What Would Gabby Say?

Gabrielle Elise Jimenez

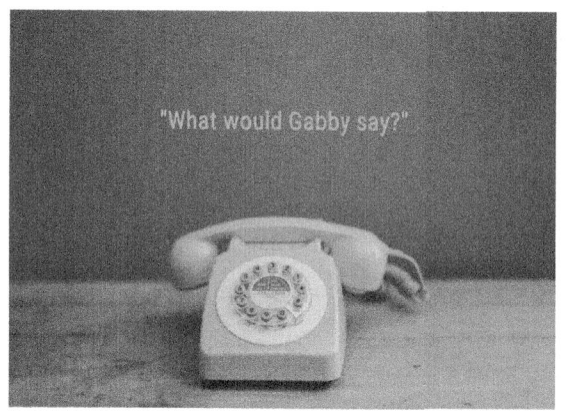

This book is dedicated to the beautiful and compassionate Hospice Heart community. I have watched you offer comfort and support to complete strangers. I have seen your fear and your vulnerability. And I have witnessed your deep desire to provide care to someone who is dying. I thank you for sharing your questions and curiosities with me, and for always being open to education, change, doing this work better, and being willing to inspire a culture that wants to help improve the way human beings are cared for when they die.

I appreciate you all so much.
This book is for you, and because of you.

Xo
Gabby

I receive a lot of email and messages from the Hospice Heart FB community. Most are questions about the way someone they love is being cared for at the end of life, many are asking for clarity relative to the many misconceptions people might have about death and dying. Some need to know they did right by someone they love, some ask for tools so they can provide care, and many want to know how to do this work. I answer every message, every email, and every comment to the best of my ability.

I received an email titled, "What would Gabby say?" and that is how this started. I created a column of sorts on the Hospice Heart Facebook page where I would publicly answer the questions I received. I understand there can be many versions of answers to one question, and I never assume I am right, and others are wrong. I am always learning; I do not know it all. So, when asked these questions, I do it in the way that makes most sense to me and stays true to how I feel, and how I provide care and support to people who are dying, and those who are saying goodbye to them.

This book is a collection of the questions I have received, and my answers to them. I hope it provides you with the comfort and support you need to care for someone who is dying.

I believe that anyone who sits at the bedside of someone who is dying has a kind and compassionate heart, you are my people and I love you!!!

Xo
Gabby

Table of Contents

Pg. 6   When should we start hospice?

Pg. 8   What is a death doula?

Pg. 12 Regrets at the end of life.

Pg. 14 Transitioning vs. Actively Dying.

Pg. 16 What does it mean when 1-2 tears fall from their eye at death?

Pg. 17 Do our own emotions when someone is dying, effect how peaceful they go?

Pg. 18 When will my grief end?

Pg. 19 How to comfort someone who is grieving when you are as well.

Pg. 21 Hospice, morphine, and death.

Pg. 24 Medications given at the end of life.

Pg. 26 Does hospice provide in-home caregivers?

Pg. 29 Hospice is NOT the boss of you.

Pg. 31 Being there for someone who makes end-of-life choices you do not support.

Pg. 34 When family members don't always agree on the plan of care.

Pg. 36 Difficult deaths.

Pg. 39 Why do people hold on at the end?

Pg. 41 Fearing Death.

Pg. 43 Why do people suddenly die when you move them?

Pg. 44 Food and water at the end of life.

Pg. 46 Food is love. How to accept that at the end of life, it is not helping.

Pg. 48 As an ICU nurse what can I do to help our patients and families?

Pg. 50 The "Death Rattle"

Pg. 52 What can I say to comfort someone who is caring for a loved one that is dying?

Pg. 54 **Poem:** Sadness is woven deep inside of me

When should we start hospice?

Q.

Dear Gabby,

My mom was just told that she only has a few months left to live, maybe longer, but that is uncertain. The doctor said she should start on hospice, but I am afraid that will just make her die faster. Hospice is where people go to die, and I don't want her to feel like I have given up hope or that I want her to die sooner. How long can I wait to start her on hospice?

A.

Dear…

The first thing I want to tell you, is that you should not wait to start her on hospice. I know this is hard for you and for her but trust me when I tell you that starting her on hospice does not shorten her time, in fact, I truly believe it gives her a little more quality to the time she does have left. If you start her now, a team can come together to support her, they can be there to address any symptoms or changes she might experience.

I always wish for people to start hospice sooner rather than later for many reasons. Some people wait until they are days away from dying, after dealing with weeks or months of pain and suffering, and I know in my heart that if they started sooner, we could have found a way to reduce the discomfort to allow them a little more peace in whatever time they have left. Many times, I will meet a patient a few days, sometimes even hours, before they die, and I see their family broken from the exhaustion and heartache. If only they came on sooner, we could have helped them in so many ways.

I see so many families having a difficult time caring for their dying loved one; not having the tools or education, and not knowing how to provide care. But we do, that is what we do, and why we are here for you. We know what to do, we know how to manage symptoms, we have the tools and the team to help you navigate this difficult time.

Starting hospice sooner does not mean you are giving up hope, we encourage hope, and we want you and your mom to feel supported. Everything we do, is set with the intention of making the dying and grieving process a little less stressful, a little less painful, and always done with compassion and kindness. You deserve that and so does your mother.

Sometimes people can come off hospice because their symptoms were managed and their disease process was made more tolerable, allowing them to have more time. This doesn't happen often, but it does happen, and it is a good example of the kind of care you can receive when you are on hospice. It may not lengthen your time, but it will bring you the support, the comfort, and the care that every human being deserves to have when they are dying.

What is a death doula?

Q.

Dear Gabby,

I have watched you speak a few times and I have read all your blogs. I know you are a death doula and I think that might be something I would want to do, but I think it would also be good for my brother who will be going on hospice soon. I honestly don't even know what they do or what one is, or how to become one. Can you help me with this?

A.

Dear…

When I first decided to go back to school to become a nurse, it was with the intention of working in hospice. I had no doubt in my mind this was what I wanted to do. As a hospice nurse I provide care to someone who is dying. Over the years I have learned so much from so many people, each offering little nuggets that have molded me into the nurse I am today. But as a hospice nurse, I have protocols to follow that limit the time I can spend with patients, which does not allow for me to check in on the families after someone dies. I struggle with this.

When I first heard about the doula's I was in awe of their ability to be so incredibly present for someone who is dying, and envious that they could start with them at diagnosis, walk alongside them on their journey, be there for their death, and support those who said goodbye for as long as needed. I wanted to take what I was already doing to a deeper, and more intimate level.

It is important to note that a doula is non-medical, whether you are clinically trained or not. I am a nurse, but as a doula I cannot act as a nurse. There are boundaries and lines that I must be mindful and respectful of.

I researched many different courses and ended up receiving my certification and training, through the Conscious Dying Institute, whom I would highly recommend. This training was deep, and beautifully spiritual and taught me things about myself that both pleased and surprised me. It was probably the best thing I could have ever done for myself relative to this work and how I want to care for someone who is dying.

What is a doula? I think a doula is a companion, a guide, someone who takes your hand and lets you know that you are not alone and will offer you comfort and support as you go through the process of dying. A doula helps you to choreograph a death that honors your wishes, that is designed by you, for you. A doula understands what it means to hold space for someone else, to be fully present for another, and to show up.

Most hospices do not have a doula on their team, as this would not be covered under the hospice benefit. I have heard that some hospices do have doulas, but I think they either pay them out of pocket, or they are volunteers. I think that a doula would be a benefit to the patient, the family, and the hospice team. I also think they would help to fill gaps which happen due to staffing shortages, high patient loads and time constraints. For now, I bring what I have learned as a doula into my work as a hospice nurse and I think that it has made me a better nurse.

As a doula you can create your own "package" of what you are able to offer, and what you want to charge. Some provide comfort and support, some provide education, some provide end-of-life planning and helping with Advance Directives and filling out legal paperwork, some provide it all. I focus mainly on education, handing over tools, preparing a patient and family, and I also really enjoy planning beautiful and unique end-of-life ceremonies and celebrations of life. I include many rituals and ceremonies in my work, helping people to find peace, to let go of weight they have been carrying, to find beautiful ways to say goodbye and to soften the grief journey if possible.

If you do not have any experience in end-of-life care, and if you have never sat at the bedside of someone who was dying, my advice would be that you take the hospice volunteer training and do that work. Their teaching is incredible, and, in my opinion, hospice volunteers are doulas without the certificate.

One day I hope to see doulas as a member of the hospice team, because I truly believe it would benefit everyone. And if that is not possible, then at the very least, have each member of the team trained to be doulas.

***I know that social workers refer caregivers to families, perhaps they could also refer doulas. Let's start there. If they cannot be a part of the team, what if they could offer the family a little more support, someone that could work with the team, and be there for the patient and the family. There are many ways this could work and benefit everyone involved.

I advise you to research several doula programs to find the one that speaks to you. While a weekend course can offer you a certificate, it doesn't necessarily make you a doula. The in-depth training from the longer courses is beneficial, so is having bedside experience. To be a doula and to truly be able to do this work, takes time, set with intention. Don't rush through this, take your time, do the work, gain experience. It is all about trust and that needs to be earned.

Regrets at the end of life.

Q.

Dear Gabby,

My dad is on hospice and only has about a week left. He keeps telling me that he has so many regrets. I want to tell him he has nothing to regret, because I think he has lived a full life, but I feel like I can't say that to him. I want to help him somehow. I also worry that I might feel the same way when it is my time to go, I already feel regretful. Why do people suddenly have so many regrets just before they die?

A.

Dear…

One of the things I witness often, is the sudden realization of how much was not said or done, when a timeframe is placed on life. Time takes on a new meaning, you wish you had more, you wish you did and said more, and most people regret that they kept putting off so much. So, when someone you love is dying and they tell you of their regrets, there isn't anything that you can say that would relieve them of how they are feeling.

I think the best thing you can do for your dad, is to ask him about his regrets, ask him what he would do differently if given more time. Ask him if there is any unfinished business you could take care of for him, or any messages you could pass on. But also encourage him not to focus on what he didn't or won't get to do. Sitting with that regret won't change a thing and it can waste the time that he does have left, especially the time he has left with you. Remind him of the things he has done in his lifetime, and some of your favorite memories of times you shared together.

I think you can tell him that he shouldn't have any regrets, and that from your perspective, he has had a full life that involved you and you will be forever thankful for that.

Those of us who work in end-of-life care have a habit of trying to encourage people to live their lives now, to do and say, "the things," now, and to not wait for the bedside to try and make up for lost time.

Most of the regrets I have heard are:
"I wish I had stayed in better touch with friends/family."
"I wish I traveled more."
"I wish I had tried harder to be happier."
"I wish I didn't stay in that relationship."
"I wish I had a better relationship with my kids."

My advice is that we all take other people's regrets as a reminder to live our own lives fuller, and better, so that when we find ourselves in that bed with a less than favorable amount of time left, we are not focused on what we didn't do, and instead revel in the memories of a life well lived.

You asked why people at the end of life always have so many regrets… I want you to know that not everybody has regrets. But imagine you were told today that you only had a week left; is there a list of things you wish you had done? There is no better time than right now to start removing the items off your list.

"The trouble is you think you have time."
By Jack Kornfield

Transitioning vs. Actively Dying.

Q.

Dear Gabby,

I am a hospice nurse and I really have a hard time with understanding the difference between transitioning and actively dying, and what the time frame is in between. Can you explain this to me in a way that would help me explain it to families?

A.

Dear…

I have a hard time with this as well and have found that I tend not to use words like "transitioning" except for in my charting or when updating the hospice team. Families are already struggling with so much, so I try to just say it like it is, "their body is shutting down rather quickly and at this time it could be very soon that they will begin the actively dying process." Transitioning does not have a simple timeframe to follow, it could be so many things and look so many ways. Sometimes the window between transitioning and actively dying is so small it is hard to determine one from the other. When someone is starting to withdraw, they are eating less and sleeping more, that indicates to me that they are "transitioning." I explain to the families that this is when the body has truly succumbed to the disease and is preparing itself to die.

I see the actively dying stage as when their breathing changes, when there are skin color/temperature changes, when they become less responsive, and when they sleep until they die. All of this could happen, and none of it could happen. The only predictable thing about how someone dies, is that they will die.

Timeframes cannot be predicted, and symptoms cannot be predicted. That is why you will oftentimes hear us say, "hours to days," when suggesting how much time someone has. I always try to have them prepare for sooner rather than later.

I looked up what transitioning means in hospice: "Transitioning is a very specific term in hospice care. It refers to **the final stages of a person's life**. It is recognized by trained hospice personnel by the changes in a patient's body that signal that the patient is likely approaching death within a few hours to days." *That is how I define actively dying, so there lies the confusion I experience.*

When someone has a terminal illness and starts hospice, it means that they have a limited time left. I see the whole dying process as a transition, so when decline happens, when their normal way of living begins to fade, they are transitioning. And when they start to shut down, and their breath changes, they begin to let go… and to me, that is actively dying, and it could last hours to days.

Please note that this is just my explanation. There are so many ways we can say things to a family member, and I always try to say the things that are most honest, most clear, and always gentle and compassionate. Calling it transitioning or actively dying does not change the outcome. What matters most to me, is how prepared the family is, and how comforted and supported they feel when that last breath is taken.

What does it mean when 1-2 tears fall from their eye at death?

Q.
When my mother was dying, I saw one tear coming from her right eye. I can't help but think that she was sad to go. Someone told me that people cry when they die, is that true? Was she sad?

A.
Dear …
Excellent question. In fact, I just heard Barbara Karnes talk about this as well. To be honest, I always thought that they were tears, and perhaps they were sad, and crying. I looked it up and found this: "This phenomenon known as lacrima mortis, or the tear of death is a source of mystery that transcends this mortal realm." I have also read that it is part of the body's reaction to dying, so I believe it is "normal" vs. "emotional."

However, having said that, the next time I see a tear falling down the cheek of someone who is dying, I am going to think it represents love; their love for us, and the love they know we feel for them. I do not believe that last tear necessarily represents sadness, and it is not meant as punishment, or something to leave you feeling guilty, so please remove that from the way you think or feel. I think I will just let that tear remind me that I am loved... and I hope it does the same for you.

Do our own emotions when someone is dying, effect how peaceful they go?

Q.

Dear Gabby,

It's been 21 years since my dad passed. My mom, and all my siblings were at his side. My mom was hysterical, crying, begging my dad not to go, screaming. Of course, she was devastated and distraught. But I've always wondered if my dad went peacefully. Did he have a hard time crossing over because my mom was begging him to stay? I feel he didn't have a quiet, peaceful, calm transition and it upsets me.

Thank you.

A.

Dear …

This is a wonderful question. I do think people struggle with letting go when the people they love are having a difficult time saying goodbye, but I honestly do not think they take that with them. I do think it is easier for them to really give in and let the process go smoother, when people are less emotional or reactive, however I think people need to feel whatever they are feeling. Your mom probably needed that reaction, she needed to let those emotions go and maybe she even needed him to know how hard this was for her. I think people think they need to keep their feelings in... I say... tell them everything, even the tough stuff. Once he let go, when that last breath was taken, I truly believe the rest of his journey was peaceful and beautiful. I want you to trust that.

When will my grief end?

Q

Hi Gabby,

I am having a very difficult time right now. I've lost my mom, my grandmother, and my sister in the past year. When will my grief end?

A.

Dear …

I want you to know that you are not alone. I feel you.

That is a lot of loss in such a short amount of time. Please know that I am sending your heart a lot of love.

What I have learned, from my own experience, is that grief doesn't end, and our first mistake is waiting for that to happen. It doesn't magically just go away. I have also learned that it changes over time. I have some Buddhist prayer flags in my back yard, which were brightly colored when I first got them. Over time they faded, almost to the point that I cannot see the colors or designs anymore, but I won't take them down because they are still just as brightly colored in my mind and heart and what they represent is still very powerful to me. That is what I think grieving for someone you love is. The colors of the grief will fade but we keep our love for them bright and vibrant in our hearts forever.

Take care of you. Talk about them. Take whatever time you need to feel everything you are feeling and honor that. The weight of your grief will lighten, the steps will become easier to take, and in time your pain and ache will fade… but your love for them will forever stay bright and vibrant in your heart. Trust that. Grief doesn't end, but it does become a little easier over time.

How to comfort someone who is grieving when you are as well.

Q.

Dear Gabby,

I have been reading your posts lately, which have everything to do with grief and grieving. I am experiencing all of that right now. Everything you listed is everything I feel. It has been a tough road, and I am barely getting my head above water. My best friend has been my rock, she has been there for me every day, she has come to my house, fed and bathed me, sat at my bedside and held my hand when all I could do was cry. She has been the reason I can get out of bed now.

Two days ago, her mother died suddenly. She called me to tell me and of course I expressed my condolences, but I was numb. I didn't offer to be there, I didn't rush to her side, part of me even wondered if she wasn't going to be there for me anymore and I felt angry. I hated that side of me. I have sent messages, but she has not responded. What do I do?

A.

Dear ...

The question here is how you can support someone else through their grief when you are still trying to navigate your own, and that is a valid question. I have never been in your shoes, so I am just drawing from what I think I would want.

She may or may not need you in the way that you needed her, as we all grieve differently, however my advice would be for you to think about how it felt when she was there for you and find a way to do the same for her. Show up at her door with food or wine or whatever you think she enjoys and give her the best hug she has ever received. Start there.

Ask her how you can help her, ask her what she needs. Listen to her, without bringing up your own experiences, you cannot compare grief, but you can sympathize.

She knows you know how she is feeling. Give her back some of what she gave you and when you meet in the middle, you will find a way to support each other. And when you feel the time is right, apologize for how you reacted initially, tell her how hard that was for you, be honest, be vulnerable, be her friend. And together, my hope is that you two will come out of this stronger than before.

Hospice, Morphine and Death.

I hear this question/comment very often...

Please know that I am in no way trying to change your mind, correct you, ignore your own personal experience, or downplay your feelings or opinions. I come from a perspective of a hospice nurse... your feelings are valid, I am just going to share mine.

Q.

Hi Gabby,

My dad is sick, and everyone tells me I should put him on hospice but all I hear about hospice is that people are killed with Morphine as soon as they start service. Is this true?

A.

Dear ...

I want to answer this in a way that reassures and comforts you, but it is a tough question because I know many people have not had the kind of experience I wish they did, which is exactly why you have heard this.

When someone is given a diagnosis of six months or less to live, hospice is suggested. Personally, I wish people would come on at that first diagnosis because I think they would get better care for longer, but unfortunately many will wait for those very last few days or hours.

Hospice is not a diagnosis, it is a plan of care for a diagnosis. Hospice comes with a collaborative team that provides support, education, and the tools to help you and those you love, navigate the dying process.

Do people die when they come on hospice? Yes.

Can they come off hospice? Yes

Do they die sooner because they came on hospice? No. They die when their bodies begin to shut down because of what the disease process is doing.

Morphine is one of the medications that is used, and I believe that it can be very effective. I prefer to first see if there are other ways to calm distress if possible, such as with verbal or tactile stimuli, or repositioning, but sometimes medication is the only way to tap into the symptoms someone experiences when they are dying.

Can someone die after Morphine is given? Yes.

But as I have said before, the way I look at it, is that the Morphine (or other medications) is the only language the body understands when it is suffering, it is as though it has given permission to the body to finally give in and let go. Sometimes these medications are the difference between pain and peaceful.

I know that many of you have not had the kind of care they hoped for when their loved one came on hospice, and I am so sorry about that. This breaks my heart every time I hear it. I do not believe it is a hospice thing though, and more of a facility/staff/individual thing, which makes me fight even harder to educate people who provide end-of-life care so that we can improve the way people are cared for when they die.

I am honored to work with a team of people who do provide beautiful care, and I often hear stories of other hospice workers who provide incredible care, so I know that most people ARE cared for well and I love that.

If you do not feel that the care you are given meets your approval, fight to have that changed. You are your loved one's advocate… scream to anyone who will listen and demand that they are cared for better. I need to believe that you will be heard.

I am a hospice nurse, and I know I am not the only one who cares for their patients as though they are someone I know and love personally… so please trust that your loved one will be cared for well.

Medications given at the end of life.

Same question(s) asked/answered a little differently.

Q. My mother was given Morphine and she died after that. Did the medication kill her?

Q. The hospice company my sister is at wants to give her Methadone, but I am afraid she will become addicted. Will she become addicted if they start her on this?

Q. Do the medications given at the end of life, like Morphine, Lorazepam, Haloperidol, or Methadone hasten death?

A.
I want to start by saying that I am not a big fan of pushing medications too quickly. I prefer to first try and find other ways to offer relief if possible. However, having said that, I think it is important to have medications on hand, and to educate patients and families on the benefits of the medications, and relieve them of fear. Fear plays a big role in the resistance of using the medications and I always want to remove that if possible.

When someone is given a terminal diagnosis, whether they are on hospice or not, it is already predetermined that they could die. When there is suffering of any kind, physical or emotional, the medications can bring relief. If non-pharmaceutical measures are taken, and are not effective, I would encourage you to try the medications.

Could someone die after taking them. Yes. But at least in my experience, it is not because of the medications. The diagnosis and the disease process were already ending their life. The medications calm the distress in such a way that it allows the body to shut down a little gentler, almost giving it permission to let go, and allowing them to die a little more peacefully.

Can someone become addicted to these medications? My answer is always this... if they are dying, and these medications are helping, take addiction off the table.

When someone you love is dying, and there is pain, shortness of breath, agitation, restlessness, or fear... the medications can almost always reduce the suffering and that would be my first goal.

Before I suggest medications to a patient or family, I educate them. I tell them what each medication can do, the benefits it might bring, and the way it comforts a body that is in distress.

Comfort, support, education, and the removal of fear... these are my goals ALWAYS.

Does hospice provide in-home caregivers?

Q.

My mom started on hospice, and I just found out that they will not be providing caregivers. I am so upset and do not know what to do. I feel like I was promised something I am not going to get, should I try another hospice agency?

A.

Dear …

I hear this a lot and I am constantly trying to find a way to get the information out there of what hospice does and does not provide. Hospice does provide a lot. I will tell you that hospice does not (usually) provide in-home full-time caregivers. Hospice does provide a social worker who comes to you with many resources, one of which will be a list of caregiving services that they recommend. Caregiving would come out of pocket. Your social worker can also help you with finding respite care, which can sometimes be provided through your insurance, and help with researching financial assistance, and/or resources that are affordable and available to you. Hospice also offers volunteers, which can come sit with the patient a few hours each week for 1-2 hours at a time. Even those small breaks are helpful, and this is something that is no cost to you and brings much comfort.

I have created a list of what most hospice's cover. (Not all hospices supply these items, so you would need to communicate with your team)

Medical equipment: hospital bed, bedside table, bedside commode, shower bench, wheelchair, walker, Hoyer lift, oxygen concentrator, portable oxygen tanks, nebulizer, and a suction machine.

Medications: Usually hospice only covers the symptom relief kit and medications related to the diagnosis. All other medications would need to be discussed with your case manager and Doctor.

Incontinent supplies: Diapers, diaper liners/poise pads, wipes, disposable bed protectors (chux), and gloves. Some also provide bathing cleansers, zinc-based creams/skin protectors, lotions, and mouth care supplies. Please note not all brands of supplies are provided, so if there is something specific you might want, it would be out of pocket.

Wound care supplies: Most, but not all, wound care supplies are provided.

Hospice Team: (not all hospices have the same availability)
Your doctor can come if needed but is available to you and will communicate with the team.
Your case manager will come once a week for about an hour, more often if needed.
If your case manager is unavailable, a visiting nurse can make the visit.
Your social worker can come once a week for about an hour, more often if needed.
Your spiritual counselor can come once a week, for about an hour, more often if needed.
Your home health aide can come a few times a week for bathing and are usually only there 1-2 hours, which is determined at admission, or during visits with your case manager.
A volunteer Is someone that usually comes 1-2 times a week, for 1-2 hours. You can discuss this with your social worker or case manager.

Most hospices offer a 24/7 triage line that will connect you directly to a nurse who can assist you with questions relative to your care and send a nurse if needed.

Not all hospices are the same, some offer more than others, and some offer different schedules and availability.

I hope this information is helpful.

Always reach out to your team and ask the questions. Hospice is a team that collaborates to ensure that you and your loved one are provided with the care, education, and tools to better navigate the end-of-life journey. Never hesitate to ask, and if we don't have the answer, we will find someone who does. We are here for you and want you to feel well supported.

Hospice is NOT the boss of you.

Q.

Dear Gabby,

Our dad was on hospice, and we are not happy with what we received. Our nurse barely communicated with us, we felt like we were held captive by them, they made all the decisions, and we had no idea whether or not what they were suggesting, was in his best interest or not. I have read all of your posts and I feel like what you provide is not what we received. I want to know what we could have done differently.

A.

Dear…

It always saddens me when I hear someone say they did not receive good care while their loved one was on hospice. Following a comment like that, the three things I hear most frequently are lack of communication, team member was not a good fit, or they were not prepared/educated/guided for what the decline would look like, or how soon it would/could happen.

I will start by saying that hospice is not the boss of you. I cannot speak for everyone else out there, so I will simply come from my own personal perspective. I think we do the very best that we can, and sometimes, admittedly, we are short staffed and might not be able to offer the time a family needs, and I struggle with that because I want to be able to offer more. And while I think I am a good hospice nurse; I have experienced a family not wanting me there. It hurt my feelings, but I had to remind myself that this is not about me, and each patient and family needs to feel safe, secure, and trusting of the people that are there to support them.

We cannot fix something we do not know is broken. You are their voice, and you have every right to complain to us, to ask for more information, for better communication, and even to change a member of your hospice team. This is not about us; this is about someone you love, and you are their advocate.
Raise your voice! Tell us what you need. Tell us what you expect(ed).

If you are uncertain about anything, or need more education about medication, or what is available to you, or what the end-of-life decline looks like, ask more questions. If you are not comfortable with your team, let them know what you are struggling with. At least give them the opportunity to address your concerns, and if that doesn't work, let them bring in someone new. We truly do want to honor your wants and wishes.

Yours is the voice that needs to be heard, you and your loved one deserve that. Hospice is not the boss of you, you are not held captive by what we think you might need or want. We come in with experience and knowledge, but we also know that what we bring, might not be what you need, so the very best thing you can do, is tell us.

I know it is not always as easy as that. I know that sometimes it just isn't a good fit. I know that sometimes the medications don't work the way we hope they do, or needs are not as addressed as they should be. Things happen. But at the end of the day, I feel confident in telling you that we truly do try to offer you everything we possibly can to help you navigate this process. Most people are not prepared for someone to die, there is a lot to understand. We have the tools, tell us what you need, want, and expect, so that we can hand the right ones over to you.

Being there for someone who makes end-of-life choices that you do not support.

Q.

Gabby,

My sister wants to take the medications that will end her life. It is legal where she lives, and she has already started the process and asked me to come be with her. I have told her many times I am not comfortable with this and will not support her wanting to kill herself. I think she needs professional help if she is feeling suicidal. This is so wrong. How can I talk her out of it.

Note: Before sending my answer, I wanted to confirm a few things; I found out that not only is she terminal, with a very short time left to live, she has also been struggling with severe unmanageable pain, that will more than likely worsen, causing her to suffer until she dies. She is also alone.

A.

Dear...

As you may know, I am an advocate for Medical Aid in Dying. I would never try to force someone to support something they were very strongly against, so please know that is not my intention.

While this might come off as harsh, please hear me out. This is not about you. You love her, and that is clear. You are worried about her, and that is important. But your sister is suffering. Will these medications end her life? Yes. But they will also end her suffering on her terms.

If there is no other option that would relieve her of this pain she is struggling with, and it is made quite clear that it will only increase, wouldn't you want to find something that could bring her comfort. Doesn't she deserve that?

I have witnessed about 50 different terminal patients take these medications, and the peace that I watch come over them, realizing their suffering is about to end, is enough for me to continue to support this choice.

As humans, we are selfish. When we love someone, we want to keep them forever. Taking these medications feels like they are being ripped away from us too soon... but isn't their diagnosis already doing that?

You do not have to agree with this choice, but at the very least, I ask that you please reach out to her, tell her you love her and if you can, please be with her when she does this. She has asked you to be there because she loves you. What she needs most of all right now is your love and support.

Choosing to take these medications is brave. It isn't about giving up, or failing, or being weak, it is about making a choice to relieve suffering that would have lingered far too long. No one wants that for someone they love.

I know this is hard, I get that. She chose you to be there... I hope you know what an honor that is. You don't have to agree... but I encourage you to be there, to love her, to support her, and you can absolutely let her know how terribly you are going to miss her... but because of you, she would not be doing this alone.

Update:

"Dear Gabby, after reading your response, I packed my car and drove the two days to be with my sister. We had a few days together, we told stories, we took pictures, we laughed, we cried, and it was the best time we ever had together. I was there when she took her medications. The doctor and nurse were so kind and gentle with her. I know what you mean when you see peace come over someone. She took the medications, she leaned back on her pillow, and I swear she was smiling. Her whole body relaxed. I knew she did the right thing for her, and it was not about me. I am sad, but I would have felt much worse if I was not there with her.

Thank you."

When family members don't always agree on the plan of care.

Q.

Dear Gabby,

We just brought my mom home with hospice, and I was wondering if you could answer a question. This was a very difficult decision, and I am struggling with it. We are of course making her as comfortable as we can. I am speaking to her and engaging in some conversation, but I am at odds with another family member who believes that will stimulate her and prolong the situation. Advice please if you can. Thank you

A.

Dear ...

Please forgive me for being blunt... but do not listen to that other person. Whether your mom has hours or days, know that talking to her, engaging with her, or even ignoring her and stepping back will not speed things up or slow things down.

Imagine that she hears, which I believe she does, and imagine if she knows where she is, what she is experiencing and who is there. Whether or not she has a voice or even shows facial reactions, I believe she hears you. If it were me, I would want her to hear my voice, to feel love until that very last breath. I would want her take-away to be that she was alive until that last breath, and treated as well as possible, knowing that she was (is) loved. She is alive... she deserves love, kindness, and compassion... keep doing what you are doing!!! I believe that all human beings deserve dignity. Talking to her and engaging her is honoring and caring for her well.

Whether someone has a voice or not, if they are at the end of their life, always assume they hear and feel. Talk to them, be respectful and gentle. Say all the things.

Difficult deaths.

Q.

Hi Gabby. I am also a hospice nurse, and I love reading your patient/family stories, which are always so beautiful. You never share the difficult ones, which I know from my own experiences, there are many. Could you share one of your hardest situations?

A.

Dear...

You are right, there are many difficult situations and I think I have even posted a blog or two relative to death being messy, and not always peaceful or beautiful. I think it is important that people know all the colors of death and dying, so I appreciate this question very much.

During the height of COVID especially, I cried almost every day and wondered if I was going to be able to continue to do this work. I sat with so many patients who were dying alone and held phones to their ears so their families could say goodbye, and it broke me. I questioned whether or not I could continue doing this work. The power of touch is such a huge part of what we do, and to not be able to do that was going against everything I believed in. This was the most difficult time for me.

I have witnessed deaths that did not go as we hoped, where the family struggled because it was too hard to watch their loved one suffer, which is what, in their eyes they were doing. Sounds and some movements can be scary. I understand that. I try to prepare everyone.

There is one story which I will never forget because it taught me so many lessons. It was several years ago when I had only just started working in hospice. I went to see a patient who had just been admitted, to check in and see how he was settling in. His wife and daughter answered the door. I asked how he was doing, and his wife said that he was sweating a lot, his skin was a different color, and he was not talking. When I walked into the room, I found him curled up in the middle of the bed, lying in a pool of sweat, and his skin was blue from his head to his feet. I had never seen anything like that before. I knew he was dead, or at least very close. His daughter asked me if I could "fix" him.

My immediate reaction was to get him repositioned in the bed, cleaned and warm, and gather his wife and kids around him to say goodbye. But his wife was not ready, and she told me to save him. She kept screaming at me to save his life. So, I did. I got him on oxygen, I gave him CPR, I had the family call 911, who came in and hooked him up to even more oxygen, and he was alive. The wife was so thankful, but I was beaten and when I went out to my car afterwards, I sobbed, and I sobbed.

He remained on life support for about 4 months, before the family was ready to let him go. I visited a few times. His wife kept thanking me, but in so many ways, I felt like I had done him a disservice.

I carried that with me until he died. I ran into my boss who asked how I was doing. I told him how I was feeling. He sat me down and he said, "Gabby, you always remind people that this is not about them. It is time you listen to your own advice." He reminded me that this was not about me.

He was dying, but his family needed to know they did everything they possibly could for him. Could I have made his landing softer? Yes. But it wasn't time for me yet. They needed more and regardless of how it made me feel, I did give them what they needed.

I am now constantly reminded that their situations, their choices, and their family dynamics are not about me. My role is to offer comfort and support in whatever way is needed. That was a tough day for me and thankfully I have never experienced anything like that again. But I learned that we cannot project our thoughts and feelings onto someone else.

I was a new nurse at that time… I think there are a few things I would do differently, but I learned from it.

Why do people hold on at the end? *I receive many versions of this question often...*

Q.

Hi Gabby, I have been sitting next to my mom's bedside for two weeks. Every day the hospice nurse tells us she is close. She has said "hours" so many times, it has now turned into weeks, and we are all wondering why she won't let go. What can we say? And I feel horrible because I am wishing she would let go. Please help me.

A.

Dear...

I often tell people it could be hours to days when I think they are close, but there have been times when I stayed a little longer so that I could be there for them, and they died four days later. It is hard enough watching someone die, preparing for that loss, and sitting vigil at their bedside, but to have someone linger for days can be frustrating, exhausting, and increase the emotions you are already feeling in a way that beats you down.

The body is a miraculous thing, and it knows what to do. And while their mind and spirit are ready to go, and perhaps have already left, the body might need more time and will linger, and there is nothing we can do about this but wait.

People ask me what they can say to help them let go. I have learned that most of what we say is more for the person who is saying goodbye, so what I usually suggest, is to say thank you, I love you and goodbye.

Lately I have suggested you find a book and start to read it a little every day. They might let go before you finish, they might hold on until the end, they may not go for another day or two, but at least you have set purpose for each day, you have prepared yourself that it might be a while, and you don't sit there watching each breath as though it was the last.

In my opinion, a terminal diagnosis lets us know that time will be shortened for someone we love, and a hospice doctor or nurse can give an estimated time frame of hours to days. But that last breath will come when the body is ready to let it go. Our job is to prepare ourselves, to make sure we have said the things, and to sit back and wait. And in the meantime, you absolutely must sleep, eat, get fresh air, and allow others to sit at the bedside for (and with) you.

And if they should happen to take that last breath when you have left the room… it's okay. You do not have to be there every second. Perhaps they wanted privacy, perhaps they didn't want that to be the last thing you saw… perhaps you had provided the words, the permission, the love, and the support enough for them to finally let go and give in to the end. And that is a beautiful thing.

Fearing Death.

Q.

Dear Gabby, I am not sick, in fact I am a very healthy 82, but I know that I do not have a lot of time left. I am starting to realize that I am afraid to die. How do I stop feeling this fear, and how can I find peace with it when that time comes?

A.

Dear ...

I am asked this a lot, usually by someone who is at the end of their life. I think most of the fear I witness comes from the unknown. While we will all take that one last breath, how we get there will differ. For some it can be in their sleep, no pain, no discomfort, no struggle. But because the other alternative is a real possibility, I think that is what breeds fear. The anticipation of there being pain or struggle can most definitely bring on fear.

I was sitting with friends one day and shared a story of a "beautiful death." One of the women that was there started to cry. She was very young, early twenties, and admitted that she was scared to die. It was because of her that I realize how differently we all view death and dying and while for some they feel peace and know that when it is time, it is time, and that is enough for them, some fear death, some anticipate suffering, some equate death to pain, which turns into fear.

While I do not practice one particular faith, I am drawn to those who do because most of them have a peace within that is accepting of death because they truly believe they will be in good hands and know where it is they are going. I envy that.

I have witnessed hundreds of very last breaths. For some they were peaceful, for some there was struggle up to the end, but when that last breath is finally taken, there is this calm that comes over someone who is dying, and despite the difficulty getting there, had finally brought them peace, and they die, peacefully.

Because of what I have witnessed, I do not fear death itself. When I die, I truly believe, with every ounce of my being, that my last breath will be taken peacefully. What I fear most is missing out. I don't want to die because I have so much more I want to do and so much more love I want to give to the people in my life. I fear missing out on all the things my family will experience. So, with that in mind, what I am trying hard to do, is make right now the very best that I can with those I love.

I cannot remove your fear, but I can tell you with confidence, that I believe your last breath will be taken peacefully. Trust that. And I want to encourage you to put the fear aside, and whether you have two weeks, two months or many years left... focus on the people you love, make as many memories as you can, and be accepting that when your time comes, it's time... and find peace with that.

Because of the work I do, I am constantly faced with my own mortality and the fragility of time. For Christmas this year, I gave each member of my immediate family a photo album, one for each of them with just our photos, and little personal notes. I wanted them to have a memory book of "us." This might sound a bit morbid, but I am now living a life that will leave memories behind... and that is the only thing I have control of... and I am okay with that.

Why do people suddenly die when you move them?

Q.

Dear Gabby,

My brother seemed to be taking forever to let go. He was not struggling; he didn't have secretions like I have heard about. I wished he would have been able to let go sooner, but I was thankful he was peaceful. The caregiver came to give him a bath, and as soon as she put the head of the bed down flat, he took a deep breath and died, just like that. Did we do that to him? Why did this happen?

A.

Dear... One of things I always let families know just before we are about to reposition someone, is that movement can initiate that last breath. I have seen it happen when the head of the bed is lowered, but also when they have been repositioned to their side as well. I don't have the scientific explanation as to why this happens, but from what I have witnessed, movement, especially if the person has been in one position for a long time, seems to loosen things up.

I know this might sound silly, but it's almost as though there is a blockage of sorts, something putting that person on hold, and when movement happens, the blockage is released, and they pass rather quickly. There is no harm done, you didn't hurt him in any way, you just did what his body needed, to be able to finally let go.

Food and water at the end of life.

Q.

Do people need food/water at the end of life?

A.

Dear...

When someone is actively dying, food/hydration can make it harder for the body to shut down and let go and can cause physical discomfort. In hospice, we do not hold food or fluids back, we never refuse anyone who wants to eat or drink, but we do educate families on the discomfort this would cause someone who is dying if food or hydration is forced. There will come a time during the dying process that your hospice doctor or nurse will suggest you not force someone to eat or drink, but I can assure you we would never do it if we thought that would cause any suffering.

If someone refuses food or hydration, my advice would be to honor this. There is a reason why they are refusing, which could be physical discomfort, lack of interest, and most often fear of choking due to not being able to swallow. Not eating or drinking in those last days is not going to end their life, that is already happening. The kindest and most compassionate thing we can do is to not force food or liquids in those last days. It is not helping them in any way and will not bring them comfort.

Food and hydration are a necessity for a healthy human body, but when the body is dying, it can make their dying experience much worse. If they don't ask for it, or they refuse it, do not give it.

My hope is that you know that you are not hurting them by not giving them food or liquids in those last days. In many ways you are helping and comforting them. I hope this helps clear up any confusion or worries you might have.

Food is love. How to accept that at the end of life, it is not helping.

Q.

Dear Gabby,

My mom and dad have been together seventy years and she has been preparing his meals for him for seventy years. Feeding him is her way of showing him how much she loves him, much like eating her meals is his way of saying he knows. But he is not doing well, his time is limited, and he struggles with eating. Sometimes he refuses and she doesn't like it and gets mad. She almost forces him to eat. What can I say to her to get her to stop?

A.

Dear...

This is a very common issue, and a struggle for families, for caregivers, and for anyone who has always counted on food to provide comfort and sustain life. Stopping eating feels like you are giving up, it feels like you are making someone else suffer, as though you are failing them somehow if you cannot feed them or talk them into eating.

I understand this is not a technical description, but this is how I try to explain it to families and caregivers. In general, as we get older, our throats tend to close a bit, making swallowing difficult. As our bodies start to shut down and decline, and if we are nearing the end of our life, not being able to swallow elicits fear. If you cannot bring food up or down, if it sits there unable to move, you feel like you are choking, sometimes it feels like you are drowning. Aspirating on food or water is scary and it is a horrible thing to experience. No one should ever have to go through that.

When someone refuses food or water, respect that. Sometimes it is only temporary, perhaps they just aren't hungry or thirsty at that time, or they no longer have a desire for food, or they are fearful of choking. You are not hurting them by not feeding them, especially at the end of their life. In fact, if someone is transitioning to actively dying, food and water can make it even more uncomfortable for the body to shut down. Feeding them in this instance is hurting them.

***When someone is dying, trust me when I tell you that they are not starving if they do not eat.

If they are not near the end of their life but they struggle with swallowing, talk to your doctor or nurse, ask about changing their diet to softer foods, or pureed, or using thickener for the liquids. The first sign I always look for is coughing after drinking water or when using a straw (straws tend to bring up more liquid than they can tolerate). Take a longer time in between bites and make the bites smaller, this helps too.

With regard to your mom, she has been providing food for your dad for a very long time, this is a difficult pattern to change. Be sensitive and mindful of that and find a different approach. Gently let her know the difficulty he might be having and help her to come up with a plan that would work for him (and her) and allow this to be her choice. If it is her choice to change things, making it easier for him, it is easier for her to accept than to suddenly be told she must change a pattern she has done for seventy years. Food is love… help her to find another way to show him love, that is safer for him.

As an ICU nurse what can I do to help our patients and families?

Q.

Hi Gabby, I have been following your posts for a while now and they have really helped me. I was very drawn to your recent experience with your brother in the ICU. I am an ICU nurse and while I was reading everything you went through day after day, I wondered what I could do differently, or better. I feel like you gained a lot of lessons for your work as a hospice nurse. I am not a hospice nurse, but we have many people that die in the ICU and many people we watch say goodbye. What can I do or say that can help them?

A.

Dear...

This is a fabulous question, and I am so honored you have asked this and my heart smiles that you did. I think the most important thing for us ALL to remember is that when someone is sick or dying in a bed, whether they have a room full of family, or they are all alone... they are a human being going through a difficult time and there is fear, uncertainty, sadness, and a myriad of emotions that make people feel alone.

Whether they can verbalize their needs or not, always talk to them, not over or about them.

Honor their space. That room is their home. Honor it. Ask permission to touch them. And if they cannot respond, let them know what you are doing, always. For instance: "I am about to move your pillow." They deserve to know what is being done to, and around them always.

Talk to them... say hello, let them know who you are, remind them they are a human being with feelings and that while they might be dying, they are not dead yet. Find ways to allow them to communicate and use their voice, whether it is nodding their head, or squeezing a hand. ALWAYS find a way to give them a voice, and if they don't have one, be theirs, and advocate for them.

For the family... check in often. Instead of asking how they are, simply ask if they need anything. And ask them about the human being lying in the bed. Allow them the opportunity to share the things they love about them. Give them permission to feel and share. And if they want to be alone, respect that and leave the room.

I believe that human beings deserve kindness, compassion, and respect. If you are caring for someone, remember they are human; make sure they are clean, cared for well, comfortable, and never ignored. Never ignore anyone. It is rude and unkind.

Let's help improve the way human beings are cared for!!!

The "Death Rattle"

I get asked about this a lot. (Note that the "death rattle" doesn't always happen)

I want to (in my terms) explain the "death rattle", which by the way I think is an awful term, and I wish they would call it something else. I have come to believe that it bothers us more than them. It usually happens at the end of life because our ability to swallow is reduced and we are unable to cough or bring secretions (saliva/phlegm) up or down so it hovers there and will sometimes make a loud vibrating sound, that sounds like rattling, or gurgling. Please do not rush to get a suction machine or medications like Atropine. First try to reposition them on their side. Sometimes, that alone can move the secretions just enough to quiet the noise... which again bothers us more than them. Repositioning is oftentimes the remedy.

If the secretions are filling their mouth, even spilling out, a suction machine is useful, but I want you to imagine what it must be like for the person lying in the bed. The noise is awful, but the suctioning tool is so uncomfortable, and when you are dying, that is the last thing you want happening to you. Try and use mouth swabs to remove the secretions manually first... please... it is so much gentler and far kinder. Medications like Atropine are effective, but usually more effective when the secretions are pooling in the mouth. A suction machine is also helpful in that same way. Neither are very helpful when the secretions are down the throat and just hovering there. Therefore, I believe repositioning is the best first thing to try.

My hope in sharing some of these tips/tools is to relieve your fear, and to help you be better prepared for what happens when we die. To be present for someone when they are dying, means to witness the ways our bodies shut down. It can be messy; it can even be a little scary… but our bodies know what to do and the things we experience are a natural part of the dying process.

Sometimes, I just lean in… I place my hand on their back and rub it gently, whispering… "it's okay, I am right here… I got you… you are not alone." And that… comforts them. Trust your words, your heart, and your touch… it is amazing what comfort these can bring.

What can I say to comfort someone who is caring for a loved one that is dying? How can I not take it personally when my friend doesn't have time for me?

Q.

Hi Gabby,

My friend is caring for her husband who is dying. We used to spend a lot of time together, spending at least two days a week walking or having dinner. When her husband became ill, she needed to stay closer to home, which I understood, and now that he is dying, she never leaves the house. I want to help her, but sometimes she doesn't even return my calls or text messages. I feel like a bad friend because my feelings are hurt, but I also feel like I am not there for her. How can I help her, what can I say to her, or do for her?

A.

Dear ...

When someone you love is dying, it is as though the rest of the world and everything around you, has completely disappeared, and all you can think about is the millions of things you need to do for them. And when you hear the phone ring or see a message pop up, all you can think about is that you will have to get back to them later. And "later" becomes a whole lot longer than you intended.

I can only speak for myself, but when I have been in this situation, I felt like I needed to be there 24/7, taking on all the tasks, even if help was offered. It is really hard to pull away, even harder to justify taking time out for yourself. And no matter how exhausted you might be, you get up the next morning and do it all over again.

Trust me when I tell you that your friend is comforted by your messages… keep them coming.

Imagine your friendship, the way it used to be, is on pause for now. Give your friend the space she needs, check in often, and if/when she reaches out to you, be there. And don't take it personally. It isn't personal.

Offering food to someone who is stretched thin, is always a good idea. Send her a message, and rather than asking her what she might want, tell her the restaurant/deli/store you will be going to and list four items she can choose from. Don't make her work too hard, meet her halfway; *"Hi friend, I am at Joe's Diner and want to bring you dinner… would you like a burger, a steak, a salad, or pasta?"* She might say no, but what if she doesn't? The dynamics in your friendship might change but there is usually a way to change with it, and again, meet her halfway.

Remember that this is not about you, even if you are having a reaction to it all. She needs to be where she is right now, doing what she is doing, and stepping away from that, regardless of how healthy it might be for her, is not a choice for her at that moment. Be patient with her, love her, let her know you are there… and don't give up on her.

Sadness is woven deep inside of me
A poem I wrote about my own grief…

I woke up early this morning
With the reminder that you are no longer here
I felt this sudden sense of sadness
And my eyes filled up with tears
The sobs are much quieter now
As though I am keeping them to myself
It's like the ache I feel when I think of you
Is stored safely on a shelf
I can reach for it when I need to
Or pretend it isn't there
But sometimes it sneaks up on me
A reminder that my sadness is everywhere
It's in the songs that I hear playing
It's in the shows that I see
It's everything, and everywhere
It's woven deep inside of me.
Sadness stays forever
It is never going to leave
Sometimes I am okay with it
But other times I cannot breathe
As I lay in bed and cried today
I whispered out your name
I told you that I missed you
That life will never be the same
The sadness will never leave me
Nor will the love I have for you
I'll take it off the shelf again
It's what I need to do
I have to work through this
All the feelings and my pain
Tears are falling from my eyes
Like a stormy winter rain
But that for me is healing
It brings comfort from the start
In many ways, each time I cry
It's as though you are visiting from my heart
As I wipe away my tears
And take care of myself
I'll say goodbye (again) for now
And put you back upon my shelf

Dear…

Thank you for taking the time to read my book. I hope that I answered some of your questions, offered you some clarity, and helped you to feel a little more confident when caring for someone who is dying.

What I want you to remember, is that dying is something we all do, and the body knows what to do. Trust that. There will be differences in the breathing, and in the facial expressions, and there will be sounds and movement that might seem scary. Do not panic. The first thing I always do, is lean in, let them know I am there, remind them that they are not alone, and let them know they are safe. Fear can sometimes add to the reactions people have when they are dying. Remember that for most people there is so much uncertainty and unknown relative to dying, that it can cause anxiety. First try verbal or tactile stimuli, and if that doesn't work, be open to and trust the medications.

I am not one to take vital signs often, because I feel like that sets me up for failure. I encourage you to stop looking at their oxygen level or forcing blood pressure readings. If they are near death, don't put them through that, it is not comforting and will only increase their anxiety. We do not die the same way, so remember that their nailbeds will not always turn blue, their body may not become cold, and their breathing could be rapid, or unusually slow. Some will have apnea, holding their breath, but some will never have that. Some people have the "death rattle," some never do.

How someone dies is not predictable, so my advice is to be prepared for what could happen, but don't wait anxiously for any of it. The more you focus on what is or is not happening, is time wasted, when you could be more present for them.

Trust that they can hear you and say the words they might need to hear, such as "thank you," "I love you," "you matter," and "goodbye." And if they should die after you walk out of the room, it's okay… maybe they didn't want an audience, maybe they didn't want that to be your last memory. ***I truly believe that what they take with them is not who was there for the very last breath, but who was there all along.***

After the last breath is taken, reach out to the people who love you, let them be there for you, and accept the out-stretched hand. Say their name often. Celebrate their life and their death. Don't let anyone tell you how long you should grieve for. Practice self-care. Take care of you… you deserve that. And remember… you are not alone.

Xo
Gabby

*Talking about death and dying
will not make it happen any faster.*

*Please have this conversation with the people you love.
Find out what their wishes are so that when that time comes,
you can honor them in the way they deserve.*

Start with some simple questions:
Where do you want to be?
Who do you want there?
Who do you not want there?
Who do you want caring for you?
How do you want your pain managed?
Who do you want to make decisions on your behalf?
How do you feel about medications?
Do you want prayers?
Do you want to have people at your bedside?
Is there something you would like to have read to you?
Would you like music played?
Have you made a musical playlist?
Do you want to be buried or cremated?

Please visit my website for:

My blogs

Class information

Podcasts and interviews

My other books

www.thehospiceheart.net

FB: The Hospice Heart
https://www.facebook.com/thehospiceheart.net

Thank you…

xo

Gabby

Made in the USA
Monee, IL
26 April 2022